Sleep Medicine and Oral Appliance Therapy

Sleep Medicine and Oral Appliance Therapy

A MANUAL FOR PHYSICIANS AND DENTISTS

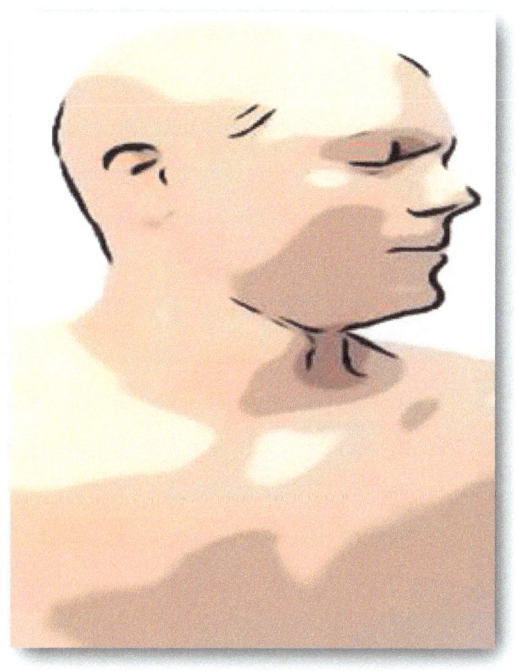

Medical Dental Guild/Amazon

Dr. Peter Chase

ISBN: 1508536988
ISBN 13: 9781508536987
Library of Congress Control Number: 2015902772
CreateSpace Independent Publishing Platform
North Charleston, South Carolina

Preface

This manual is designed for physicians and dentists wanting to explore their possible role in the field of sleep medicine and the treatment of sleep related breathing and movement disorders. In writing *Sleep Medicine and Oral Appliance Therapy*, I wanted to create a concise manual that provided essential information to medical and dental professionals.

Millions of people suffer from obstructive sleep apnea and arousal from excessive muscle activity during the sleep period. The apparent medical implications of these disorders are multiple. Sleep medicine is a growing field, and it is apparent that multiple medical specialties are essential to comprehensive diagnosis and treatment. The broadness of the field demands a team approach to optimal care.

A more comprehensive medical history and systems review is required. Providers must have a clear understanding of medical diagnostic and treatment coding with all insurance transactions done through medical insurance.

Clinical evaluation is expanded to include detailed information on the head and neck, joints and muscles, and nasopharyngeal and oropharyngeal airways. In addition, dental findings are expanded to include orthodontic and prosthodontic details. The use of CBCT imaging information is important to more completely evaluate the patient's medical and dental condition.

Sleep disorders including obstructive sleep apnea and periodic limb movement disorder are considered medical conditions, and the physician is responsible for all sleep medical diagnoses. The dentist is a provider of oral appliance therapy for obstructive sleep disorders and musculoskeletal problems involving the jaw.

Organized medicine supports physicians and dentists providing screening of their existing patients for possible sleep-related disorders. Office brochures and questionnaires are effective communication and are helpful to patients. Primary care physicians, sleep medicine specialists, and otolaryngologists are involved in patient workup and sleep-study referral. If the patient is diagnosed with airway problems or jaw related musculoskeletal problems, oral appliance therapy is a considered treatment option.

The dentist providing patient evaluation and oral appliance therapy as an aspect of medical management communicates with the physician on each step of the treatment process. Oral appliances selected should meet durable medical equipment (DME) guidelines. Referral back to the physician for follow-up sleep study assessing appliance efficacy is expected.

Enjoy the adventure!

Thank you to the Medical Dental Guild for helping support this publication.

Contents

Acknowledgments

would like to thank the following individuals for reviewing this manuscript and for making both editorial and content suggestions: psychiatrist James Gracer, MD; radiologist Shikha Rathi, DDS, MS; pulmonologist/ sleep medicine specialist Michael Cohen, MD; physical therapist Leslie Hisaka, PT; primary care physician Rebecca Parish, MD; otolaryngologist Randell Wenokur, MD; DME specialist Jim Adiago; and Aether Medical Management director Mark Bottini.

CHAPTER 1

Sleep Medicine and Sleep-Related Breathing and Movement Disorders

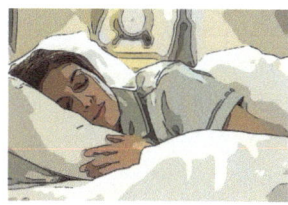

The science of sleep medicine has developed over the last sixty years. One of the first major sleep centers was created at Stanford Medical School in the 1970s, using early developments in polysomnography and positive airway pressure treatment prototypes. The American Medical Association recognized sleep medicine as a subspecialty in 1995.

Early researchers discovered that sleep was a much more complex process than previously recognized, and that there was a clear physiological difference between the waking and sleeping state. Sleep has been defined as a condition of body and mind in which the nervous system is relatively inactive, the eyes are closed, the postural muscles are relaxed, and consciousness is suspended. Different stages during the sleep period have been observed, along with variations in physiological processes. There are three recognized sleep stages of non-rapid eye movement (NREM) sleep in addition to what is called the rapid eye movement (REM) stage.

Non-REM Sleep (NREM)   REM Sleep

- Stage 1
- Stage 2
- Stage 3

In healthy sleep dynamics, the approximate ninety-minute sleep cycle (NREM stages 1–3 and REM) repeats four to six times per night. Lighter stages of sleep are stages 1 and 2, progressing to deeper sleep stage 3 (NREM) and to REM-period sleep with muscle atonia. A regular, uninterrupted sleep period appears essential to optimal daytime functioning.

Sleep Disorders

It has been estimated that nearly sixty million people in the United States suffer from irregular and interrupted sleep periods. The lack of adequate sleep has been associated with a variety of symptoms and medical issues, the most common of which is daytime fatigue. Other complaints include morning headaches, multiple night awakenings, depression, and sleep partner disruption resulting from snoring and excessive movement. Research has shown statistical correlations between sleep deprivation and cardiovascular, pulmonary, gastroenterological, neurological, endocrinological, musculoskeletal, otolaryngological, urological, and psychological abnormalities.

Although the *International Classification of Sleep Disorders, Second Edition (ICSD-2)* has classified ninety-six sleep disorders, the most commonly recognized sleep disorders are the following:

- Insomnia
- Sleep-related breathing disorders (SRBD)
- Periodic limb movement disorders (PLMD)

The primary care physician (PCP) is the clearinghouse for the medical system. With the multitude of overlapping symptoms, these physicians have a complex job in differential diagnosis. They must be alert to cardiovascular issues, glandular dysfunction, Alzheimer's disease, or any of the many diseases or disorders capable of producing symptoms similar to those from sleep-related disorders. Blood tests, stress tests, and psychological evaluations may be appropriate diagnostic tools.

If a sleep-related breathing or movement disorder is the working diagnosis, the PCP may order either a laboratory or home sleep test; negative results for a sleep-related breathing or movement disorder require further diagnostic efforts. Depending on the differential diagnosis, treatment may be directed at cognitive, neurological, hormonal, pain-related, behavioral, emotional, or musculoskeletal disorders, as well as other issues. If the patient is diagnosed with a sleep-related breathing or movement disorder, the PCP may elect to direct treatment or to refer the patient to a sleep specialist. The most common board-certified sleep physicians are pulmonologists, otolaryngologists, and neurologists. In some cases, the sleep specialist performs the primary evaluation of the patient. Treatment providers complete their own specialty evaluations.

Sleep-related breathing disorders are classified as *central* or *obstructive* in nature.

Central sleep apnea is considered a relatively rare neurological problem in which the brain fails to send proper signals to the muscles that control breathing. The recommended treatment for this is adaptive servo ventilation (ASV).

Obstructive sleep apnea refers to an airway obstruction problem in which the size of the airway is diminished because of tongue placement, tissue edema, or other anatomical variations. Weight gain, sleep posture, and aging may be additional contributing factors. Specific therapies depend on the primary diagnosis as determined by the sleep doctor and may include the following:

- Pneumatic splints (positive airway pressure/PAP)
- Intraoral postural splints (mandibular repositioning devices/MRD)
- Nasal and oropharyngeal surgery (uvulopalatopharyngoplasty/UPPP and tongue-base surgeries)
- Maxillomandibular surgery (mandibular osteotomy)

If tolerated, pneumatic splints (PAP) remain the most effective form of therapy. Innovation is continuing with new forms of treatment being developed. Currently under investigation are electrical muscle stimulator implants and oral suction devices.

Periodic limb movement disorder, while not considered a sleep-related breathing disorder, can be diagnosed from laboratory-based sleep studies, and focuses primarily on arm and leg movements associated with sleep disruption. Some sleep researchers have also looked at jaw movement and jaw-related muscle activity during sleep (bruxing/clenching) as a possible movement disorder associated with arousals.

Sleep medicine is a vast field comprising multiple medical specialists. Diagnosis of sleep medicine problems are considered medical issues and classified as medical care using *International Classification of Diseases (ICD-9/10)* and *International Classification of Sleep Disorders (ICSD-2)*. Treatment of sleep medicine disorders is also classified as medical care using *Current Procedural Terminology (CPT)* coding and *Healthcare Common Procedure Coding System (HCPCS)*. If physician diagnosis has been narrowed to obstructive sleep apnea or periodic limb movement disorder, physicians or dentists may provide treatment. Guidelines for management and care for sleep related disorders continue to grow and undergo changes as new forms of treatments are explored.

CHAPTER 2

Anatomy and Physiology

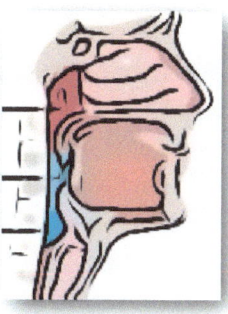

The respiratory system's primary function is to supply oxygen to all parts of the body by inhaling oxygen-rich air and exhaling carbon dioxide.

The group of tissues and organs that enable breathing includes the nose, mouth, pharynx, trachea, bronchial tubes, lungs, related muscles, and neurovascular system. The respiratory system works by breathing air in through the nose or mouth, which humidify, warm, and filter the air. The air then travels through the pharynx, down the trachea, though two main-stem bronchi (bronchial tubes), and into the lungs.

Inhalation and exhalation are the results of the diaphragm, abdominal muscles, and accessory muscles working together to expand and contract the lungs. When the air is inhaled, it goes through the bronchi in the lungs to alveoli, arterioles, and arteries. The arteries carry the blood throughout the body. With exhalation, the carbon dioxide is absorbed into the vascular system, reentering the lungs and exiting the body through the nose and mouth. If breathing is compromised, not only will the body not receive enough oxygen to keep it optimally functioning, but it will also be impaired by the carbon dioxide building up in the blood.

The airway structures involved in obstructive sleep apnea are the nose, the mouth, and the pharynx. The nasal airway extends from the anterior nostrils (nares) to the posterior nares. Clinical assessment evaluates nasal-airway patency; investigation may uncover small nares, lateral nasal collapse on inspiration, enlarged turbinate, deviated septum, nasal congestion, or other causes of nasal obstruction such as polyps.

The pharynx is a collapsible muscular tube that connects the nasal and oral cavities to the larynx and esophagus. It is common to both the alimentary and the respiratory tract.

The pharynx is divided into three sections: the nasopharynx (upper section), the oropharynx (middle section), and laryngopharynx (lower section). The entire pharynx (airway) is twelve to fourteen centimeters long (four and three-quarters to five and a half inches). The pharynx begins at the base of the skull and ends inferior to the cricoid cartilage (C6). The cervical spine makes up the posterior wall of the airway. The muscles of the pharynx are of two types:

- **Outer circular:** The outer circular muscles contract to propel bolus downward during swallowing.
- **Inner longitudinal:** The longitudinal muscles act to shorten and widen the pharynx during swallowing.

Nasopharynx

The nasopharynx is located directly behind the posterior of the nose, and extends from the base of the occipital bone downward to the upper aspect of the soft palate. It includes the salpingopharyngeus, tensor veli palatini, and levator veli palatini muscles. The nasopharynx remains open even when surrounding muscles flex to maintain respiratory function. The posterior wall of the nasopharynx contains the adenoids (pharyngeal tonsils), and the lateral wall contains the openings to the eustachian tubes, which lead to the ears.

Oropharynx

The oropharynx is located at the back of the mouth behind the oral cavity. The anterior portion includes the back third of the tongue, the soft palate, the uvula, and the epiglottis. In the lateral walls, between the palatoglossal and the palatopharyngeal arches, are the palatine tonsils. The oropharynx extends inferiorly to the level of the hyoid bone, accepting air from the nose or mouth and passing it to the laryngopharynx. The oropharynx also accepts food from the mouth and passes it to the esophagus. Soft palate muscles involved in swallowing are the tensor veli palatini, the palatoglossus, the levator veli palatini, and the musculus uvulae. The uvula is mobile, consisting of muscle fibers sheathed in mucous membrane, and is responsible for closing off the nasopharynx during swallowing.

The eight muscles of the tongue are classified as either intrinsic or extrinsic.

Four paired intrinsic muscles of the tongue originate and insert within the tongue. These muscles alter the shape of the tongue, facilitating speech, swallowing, and eating.

- Superior longitudinal
- Inferior longitudinal
- Vertical
- Transverse

The extrinsic muscles originate from bone and extend to the tongue. Their main functions are altering the tongue's position, allowing for protrusion, retraction, and side-to-side movement.

- Genioglossus—protrudes the tongue
- Hyoglossus—depresses the tongue
- Styloglossus—elevates and retracts the tongue
- Palatoglossus—elevates the back of the tongue

The mouth has multiple functions as the accessory orifice for breathing and the primary organ of communication and speech. It is the beginning of the alimentary tract and the portal for intake of food and liquids, where critical digestive functions including tasting, masticating, and swallowing take place. The salivary glands provide lubrication for swallowing and moving the food along the alimentary tract. Chewing, swallowing, and speaking involve the tongue, masticatory, cervical, and facial musculature. The paired temporomandibular joints (TMJs), which allow for jaw movement, are unique in their coordinated rotational and translational motions. In addition, the disc that separates the ball of the joint from the socket is made up of fibrocartilage, a more durable tissue than the hyaline cartilage present in other joints. The TMJs are also the only joint system to have muscles attached to both the disc and the ball of the joint.

Laryngopharynx

The laryngopharynx is the caudal portion of the pharynx, beginning at the upper portion of the epiglottis and opening into the larynx and esophagus. The lingual tonsils are located at the base of the tongue. Air, food, and fluids continue downward to the opening of the esophagus and trachea, where air enters the trachea and food and fluids flow into the esophagus. The hyoid bone is located at the base of the tongue and mandible, anterior to the epiglottis and superior to the anterior portion of the larynx. The hyoid bone and attachments are thought to be involved in sleep apnea, as they play a part in tongue posture and movement and in swallowing.

CHAPTER 3

Pathology Underlying Sleep-Related Breathing and Movement Disorders

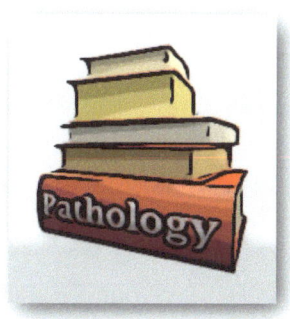

Patients who are suffering from inadequate restorative sleep may have a variety of issues affecting their sleep patterns. These issues could include psychological, environmental, and physical factors. Normally, it is the responsibility of the primary care physician (PCP) to conduct a full examination of the patient and provide a differential diagnosis. If sleep-disordered breathing or movement disorders are suspected, a comprehensive polysomnogram (PSG) is recommended. Use of home sleep testing (HST) is convenient, but is more limited in diagnostic information.

PSG information helps to identify the type of sleep apnea (obstructive, central, or mixed). It also provides data on irregularities in sleep dynamics (architecture and patterns) and arousal-related muscle activity. If the sleep test is negative for sleep apnea or movement disorder, the PCP will explore alternative diagnoses or refer the patient to a certified sleep physician for a more definitive sleep-related diagnosis.

It is generally agreed that human development is imperfect, including the area of the middle and lower face. Patients diagnosed with obstructive sleep apnea have recognizable characteristics, including retrognathia involving both the maxilla and mandible, insufficient vertical development of the maxillomandibular complex, lateral narrowing of the maxilla and mandible, narrowing of the base of the nose, and elevation of the hard palate. The result is the apnea-prone patient with limited tongue space, narrowing of the oropharyngeal airway, and compromised breathing. Abnormal muscle activity (bruxing or clenching) may also be related and considered a movement disorder associated with arousals.

Whether using positive airway pressure, oral appliances, surgical interventions, or other means to maintain an open airway during sleep, the treatment is directed at a problem that has developed over the life of the individual patient. There are other contributing factors to these disorders such as weight gain, side effects from medications, and aging. However, as medicine addresses the basis of obstructive sleep apnea and movement disorders, growth and development must be closely evaluated, and the dentist can be a helpful colleague in this investigation.

If the therapy selected is a mandibular repositioning device (MRD), the physician has decided that enhancing the environment for the tongue is the best solution for the patient. Bringing the tongue forward, increasing the vertical height between the maxilla and mandible, artificially increasing cervical muscle tone, and encouraging behavioral changes with body posture modification during sleep are treatment objectives.

Dentists trained in musculoskeletal problems involving the jaw can provide support to the physician with management of oral appliance therapy. In addition, the dentist can be helpful in collecting diagnostic obstructive sleep apnea data. Through a comprehensive clinical evaluation and sophisticated imaging, the dentist is able to provide objective data on measurements of retrognathia and maxillomandibular development. Imaging can provide cephalometric data on facial asymmetries and important skeletal dimensions. In addition, the health of the dental and periodontal supporting structures, and health of the temporomandibular joints and upper cervical spine can be documented. The joint–muscle systems of the jaw joint and upper cervical joints are what allow mandibular reposturing. And perhaps most importantly, these studies provide objective data on the size of the airway and the location of greatest restriction. Oral appliance (MRD) design varies, depending on individual patient dynamics.

With the dentist assuming a greater role in multidisciplinary care of the patient, the etiology of sleep-related breathing and musculoskeletal disorders can be better understood. The scientific data collected has the potential of changing protocol and supporting earlier treatment of high-risk patients. The general dentist and the dental specialties of pedodontics and orthodontics can take on greater responsibility in the development of the maxillomandibular complex. Facial development will be more closely scrutinized with the use of sophisticated appliances directed at facial growth and enhancement of airway and optimal muscle and joint function. Use of medical diagnostic devices such as electromyography, sonography and movement analysis is increasing. In addition, coordinated care with physical therapists and other physical medicine specialists is improving treatment outcome.

CHAPTER 4

Sleep Disorders and the Physician

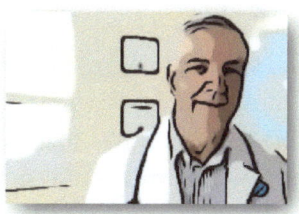

S leep disorders are considered a medical problem with specific medical coding (*International Classification of Disease* and *International Classification of Sleep Disorders: Diagnostic & Coding Manual*). Differential diagnoses may include insomnia, movement disorders, cognitive disorders, neurological disorders, hormonal disorders, pain disorders, behavioral disorders, psychological disorders, musculoskeletal disorders, biochemical disorders, or other health-related issues. Patient triage could include the primary care doctor, medical specialist, and sleep medicine specialist. The medical field is recognizing that inadequate, disrupted sleep could be the basis of a variety of medical problems including disorders involving cardiovascular, pulmonary, gastrointestinal, neurological, endocrinological, otolaryngological, urological, and musculoskeletal systems. In addition, sleep issues may be operant in chronic pain and cognitive or behavioral disorders.

Initially, patients complaining of fatigue or other possible sleep-related symptoms report their concerns to their PCP. If sleep-related breathing disorders or movement disorders are suspected, the patient may be referred to a sleep specialist. The PCP or the sleep specialist may refer the patient for a sleep study. Based on the clinical evaluation and this study, a diagnosis is made, upon which the patient may be referred for further testing or directly treated by the PCP or sleep specialist.

Medications
If the diagnosis includes periodic limb movement disorder (PLMD), the primary treatment is medication. General categories of drugs used to treat PLMD include the following:

- Dopamine agonists
- Anticonvulsants
- Benzodiazepines
- Opioids

Positive Airway Pressure (PAP)

If the diagnosis is obstructive sleep apnea (OSA), the primary treatment recommended by the physician is pneumatic splint therapy or positive airway pressure (PAP). The actual design of the PAP unit may vary between continuous positive airway pressure (PAP), oral positive airway pressure (OPAP), bilevel positive airway pressure (BiPAP), or auto-adjusting positive airway pressure (AutoPAP) depending on the needs of the patient. If PAP therapy is optimally adapted to the patient, treatment effectiveness can be as high as 90 to 95 percent reduction in OSA events. PAP treatment is also used as part of the sleep study to evaluate treatment effectiveness in resolving OSA condition.

Oral Appliance Therapy (MRD)

An alternative treatment for OSA is the oral appliance or mandibular repositioning device (MRD). The practitioner providing MRD care has a working knowledge of anatomy, the dentition, and musculoskeletal problems involving the jaw. The effectiveness of MRD therapy is less than PAP therapy; however, with improved MRD compliance, the overall success of MRD and PAP treatments may be relatively equivalent. If optimally designed, the oral appliance has been shown to reduce OSA events by approximately 75% with good compliance. The oral device is prescribed primarily for mild to moderate OSA patients where the reduction of the OSA events will bring the patient's condition closer to a normal range (zero to five events per hour). The device can also be used for more severe cases where the patient is unable to adapt to, or does not desire CPAP therapy; however, residual OSA events may remain. Combination therapy using both CPAP and an oral appliance has been shown to be effective in managing severe cases. Compliance monitoring chips are available for most oral appliance designs. Dentists may facilitate treatment progress with HST oral appliance efficacy testing or refer the patient for sleep laboratory testing.

Surgery

Additional alternative therapy includes surgeries provided by the otolaryngologist and the oral maxillofacial surgeon. If the clinical workup of the patient includes findings of large tonsils/adenoids, elongated soft palate, atypical uvula, enlarged turbinates, deviated septum or enlarged tongue, surgery is consideration. Tissue reduction and modification has been shown to be effective in reducing OSA events. In very severe cases, where less invasive therapies have not been effective, hard tissue surgery with mandibular advancement and maxillomandibular advancement may be a treatment alternative provided by the oral maxillofacial surgeon or otolaryngologist. Regardless of the treatment recommended, physicians provide information on sleep hygiene, alternative sleep postures, and pillow and bed design.

CHAPTER 5

Obstructive Sleep Disorders and the Dentist

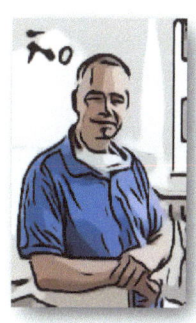

Because the obstructive sleep apnea research over the last two decades has validated the effectiveness of mandibular repositioning devices (MRD), the MRD has become a more popular prescribed alternative to PAP therapy. Historically, dentists have functioned independently of physicians, with separate training programs. Dentistry has not adopted *The International Classification of Diseases (ICD-9/10)* diagnostic coding system or the *International Classification of Sleep Disorders (ICSD-2) diagnostic system.* They also are not generally trained to use *Current Procedural Terminology (CPT)* or *Healthcare common procedure Coding System (HCPCS)* that are used by other health care providers for medical treatment coding. Unique to dentistry is the adoption of *Current Dental Terminology (CDT)*, a proprietary treatment coding system.

Unlike medicine, which primarily functions as a group practice–based, hospital-aligned profession, dentistry is primarily a solo practice–based, non-hospital-aligned profession. Dentists view themselves as responsible for diagnosing and treating dental and periodontal disease, and play a key role in facial aesthetics through orthodontics and cosmetic dentistry.

Despite the existence of nine dental subspecialties, the majority of dentists practice general dentistry, providing much of the specialty care within the general dental office. Recognized dental subspecialties include the following:

- Dental public health
- Endodontics
- Oral and maxillofacial pathology
- Oral and maxillofacial radiology
- Oral and maxillofacial surgery
- Orthodontics
- Periodontics
- Pediatric dentistry
- Prosthodontics

It is a long-standing function of both specialty and general dentistry to provide various forms of oral appliance therapy, including removable prosthetic devices for missing teeth, night guard splint therapy to protect teeth, and orthodontic appliance care to align teeth. These procedures are considered dental care with a dental diagnosis, and are generally covered by dental insurance.

The diagnosis of obstructive sleep apnea and jaw-related musculoskeletal disorders are considered medical diagnoses, and treatment is directed by the physician (MD, DO). Providing an oral appliance that alters tongue posture to avoid airway collapse is considered medical care. Qualified dentists can provide mandibular repositioning devices (MRDs) for obstructive sleep apnea and mandibular repositioning devices for jaw-related musculoskeletal disorders. These devices are considered medical care, and are generally covered under medical insurance.

This requirement for physician diagnosis and physician-directed treatment creates a conundrum for dentists, who are trained as both diagnosticians and treatment providers. The necessity for a physician diagnosis and referral is a new paradigm for the practicing dentist. Screening dental patients for possible undiagnosed snoring and obstructive sleep apnea is encouraged by both medicine and dentistry. Once identified through questionnaires and interviews, the dentist is obliged to refer the patient for workup by a physician and testing for diagnostic confirmation.

If the patient is diagnosed with snoring, it is appropriate for the dentist to treat the condition with an oral appliance. This treatment is not generally covered by insurance.

If the patient is diagnosed with obstructive sleep apnea, appropriate therapy is at the physician's discretion. PAP therapy remains the most effective therapy. Although PAP therapy is the primary modality recommended by the physician, oral appliance therapy is also considered an accepted initial therapy option for mild to moderate OSA. If PAP therapy is intolerable, oral appliance therapy (MRD) or surgical care may be advised. Oral appliance therapy, in combination with PAP therapy, is also considered as a treatment choice in severe OSA cases.

If dentists become involved in multidisciplinary care and provide oral appliance therapy, they become part of the medical team. The dentist treating obstructive sleep disorders assumes the co-management of musculoskeletal issues involving the jaw. Physical therapy or other physical medicine referrals may be appropriate.

General dental school training does not provide curricula supporting expanded care into obstructive sleep disorders or musculoskeletal issues involving the jaw. The graduating dentist has little understanding of musculoskeletal disorders. Although dentists are taught to screen for temporomandibular disorders, there is no agreed-upon therapy for these musculoskeletal issues, and there are no dental treatment codes for joint and muscle care or airway enhancement care.

Different groups in dentistry have sought specialty status in an expanded role for dentistry including oral medicine, management of jaw-related pain and temporomandibular disorders, and now management of obstructive sleep disorders. Organized dentistry has not recognized these additional specialties, but they have supported extensive postgraduate continuing education programs. Well-trained dentists in oral medicine, airway issues and musculoskeletal problems involving the jaw are important to the medical community.

A variety of postgraduate organizations have been developed to address jaw-related musculoskeletal pain and dysfunction and obstructive sleep disorders, including:

- American Academy of Orofacial Pain
- American Academy of Pain Management
- American Academy of Craniofacial Pain
- American Academy of Oral Medicine
- International College of Craniomandibular Orthopedics
- American Sleep and Breathing Academy
- American Academy of Dental Sleep Medicine
- American Association of Physiological Medicine and Dentistry
- Academy of Clinical Sleep Disorders Disciplines
- American Academy of Gnathological Orthopedics

All of the above organizations offer diplomat or fellow status for dentists that pass their certification process. Ideally, certification includes an academic component, a clinical component, a research component, and a publishing component. Proposals to expand training programs could extend dental schooling by as much as three years. This additional training would incorporate expanded education in musculoskeletal and respiratory medicine and extended courses in the orthodontic and prosthodontic fields. Although much of the necessary science underlying these disorders is already addressed at the university level, there is no indication that dental education will be expanded beyond the current four years. Currently, a small number of dental schools are offering a postgraduate sleep medicine mini-residency programs.

Working with the physician as the diagnostician and coordinator of care remains current protocol. There have been efforts at modifying this dynamic to increase the number of patients treated with oral appliance therapy.

CHAPTER 6

Sleep Medicine Testing and Imaging

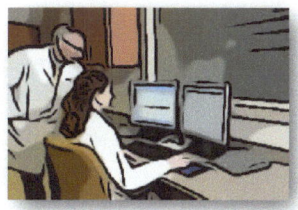

Patients may present to a physician's office with a variety of symptoms and concerns. If the differential diagnosis includes a sleep-related breathing disorder, additional evaluation is necessary to narrow the diagnosis, and to objectively support it. Sleep tests range from simple subjective questionnaires to sophisticated physiological tests.

Screening Questionnaire

These tests can be as simple as an online questionnaire or a waiting room pamphlet. Questionnaire examples are the Epworth Sleepiness Scale, the Berlin Questionnaire, the Stanford Sleepiness Scale, and the Pittsburgh Sleep Quality Index. Questions may range from inquiries about daytime sleepiness to health-related questions about breathing and sleep problems including physical, behavioral, or cognitive issues. These tests are used in conjunction with a comprehensive patient history, review of systems, and clinical examination.

Polysomnography

Testing of physiological functions is considered objective assessment. These tests range from simple, unattended single-parameter take-home studies to comprehensive multichannel laboratory studies. Except for over-the-counter, single or limited parameter tests such as pulse oximetry, sleep studies are interpreted by sleep medicine specialists.

Type I study (attended laboratory sleep study—polysomnogram/PSG)

This comprehensive study is indicated for all patients suspected of a sleep-related breathing disorder diagnosis. The Type I study monitors seven or more parameters. Additionally, this study provides objective data supporting a diagnosis of a periodic limb movement disorder (PLMD). PSG sleep studies are generally divided into thirty-second measurable periods (epochs). The sleep stage assigned to each epoch is the stage occupying the majority of time within the epoch.

Type II study (attended research-based sleep study)

This study is an attended take-home multichannel study used in sleep research.

Type III study (unattended home sleep test—HST)

This study is indicated for patients with high pretest OSA probability and without suspected comorbidities. Type III portable testing units have at least four channels (airflow, respiratory movements, heart rate, and blood-oxygen saturation). Studies have validated Type III monitoring devices with acceptable sensitivity and specificity. However, these studies are limited in physiological parameters measured, and provide less information on sleep dynamics. These studies may also be used to assess patient progress.

Type IV study (unattended home sleep test—limited)

This study is limited to one or two parameters, and is considered an inadequate sleep study. An example of this type of test is a blood-oxygen testing unit (SaO_2) that can be purchased at retail pharmacies.

Additional sleep tests:

- Multiple sleep latency test (MSLT), used as a measurement of daytime sleepiness
- Maintenance of wakefulness test (MWT), used as a measurement of daytime alertness

Sleep-testing protocols

- Brain wave activity (EEG)
- Eye movement (EOG)
- Jaw muscle activity (EMG)
- Nasal/oral airflow (catheter sensors)
- Chest/abdomen breathing effort (belt sensors)
- Snoring (digital recording)
- Heart rhythm (EKG)
- Blood-oxygen level (plethosomnogram/pulse oximetry)
- Leg muscle activity (EMG)
- Body position (digital position sensor)

Sleep staging is measured by observing characteristic electroencephalographic (EEG), electrooculographic (EOG), and electromyographic (EMG) recordings. Respiration is monitored with nasal/oral airflow (thermistors/pressure transducers) and thoracic/abdominal respiratory effort sensors. Oxygen saturation is monitored by finger oximetry. Electrocardiogram (EKG) is used to monitor cardiac rhythm.

Polysomnogram Information

1. **Apnea-hypopnea index:** apnea events plus hypopnea events divided by number of hours slept.
   OSA severity: measured AHI

   - Mild: 5–14 events per hour
   - Moderate: 15–29 events per hour
   - Severe: 30+ events per hour

2. **Arousal:** an abrupt change in brainwave activity (EEG) indicating a change from sleep to wakefulness, or from a deeper to lighter stage of sleep. A documented arousal must be greater than three seconds. Arousals may be spontaneous or related to respiratory or movement events.
3. **Arousal index:** the number of arousals per hour divided by number of hours slept. Arousals may be spontaneous or related to respiratory or movement events.

   - Normal = 0–5 per hour

4. **Blood-oxygen saturation:** level of oxygen in the blood; normal SaO2 should not go below 90 percent, or drop more than 4 percent with apnea/hypopnea event; SaO2 nadir = lowest level of blood oxygen.

   - 85–90 percent = Mild
   - 80–85 percent = Moderate
   - 80 percent or lower = Severe

5. **Cardiac abnormalities:** cardiac function abnormality with possible arrhythmia, bradycardia, and tachycardia.
6. **Central sleep apnea/hypopnea:** Interruption of oral/nasal airflow not associated with respiratory effort or airway blockage, thought to be related to a temporary irregularity in the brain's control of breathing.
7. **Central sleep apnea index:** apnea/hypopnea events that are not associated with respiratory effort.
8. **Periodic limb movement disorder:** body movements associated with arousals; could include bruxism and clenching if appropriately monitored.
9. **Periodic limb movement index:** number of body movements (skeletal muscle activity) associated with arousals per hour; normal = 0–5 per hour.

10. **REM latency:** the time it takes to obtain REM stage from sleep onset; should take between ninety and one hundred twenty minutes.
11. **REM-sleep disorder:** lack of atonia during REM sleep stage.
12. **Respiratory disturbance index (RDI):** apnea events plus hypopnea events plus respiratory effort–related arousals (RERA) divided by number of hours slept; normal = 0–5 per hour.
13. **Respiratory effort–related arousals (RERA):** arousals related to respiratory effort characterized by increasing respiratory effort for ten seconds or more leading to an arousal from sleep level, but one that does not fulfill the criteria for a hypopnea or apnea; normal = 0–5 per hour.
14. **Respiratory events (associated with arousals):** made up of obstructive apneas, obstructive hypopneas, respiratory efforts, and central and mixed apneas.
15. **Sleep apnea event:** a near to complete cessation of oral/nasal airflow not associated with respiratory effort or airway blockage; thought to be related to a temporary irregularity in the brain's control of breathing.
16. **Sleep architecture (sleep staging):** NREM stage 1 = 5 percent, NREM stage 2 = 50 percent, NREM stage 3 = 25 percent, REM = 20 percent.
17. **Sleep hypopnea event:** a partial interruption in oral/nasal airflow for then seconds or more with an accompanying decrease in blood oxygen and arousal from sleep level.
18. **Sleep efficiency:** total time spent in bed asleep (minus awakenings and how long it takes to fall back asleep) divided by the total time spent in bed; normal = 85–99 percent.
19. **Sleep latency:** length of time prior to beginning sleep; should take between ten and twenty minutes.
20. **Snoring:** measurable noise from mouth or nose during sleep; thought to be the result of diminished airway during sleep-venturi effect.
21. **Total sleep time (TST):** total period of time a patient is in bed asleep.
22. **Upper airway resistance:** breathing efforts that do not meet apnea/hypopnea standards, but are associated with arousals.

Treatment of OSA is indicated if the patient has

- an AHI/RDI greater than 15; or
- an AHI/RDI of 5–15 with symptoms or history of daytime sleepiness hypertension, stroke, ischemic heart disease, insomnia, or mood disorders.

Imaging

Panographic study

A panographic study is a routine imaging study designed for dental offices. It provides gross general pathology within the maxillomandibular structures. The panographic study, combined with dental x-rays, is appropriate for benign snoring patients with minimal health history and no history of jaw-related problems. These studies are customarily interpreted and reviewed by the dentist obtaining the study.

Cone-Beam Computed Tomography Study

The CBCT (cone-beam computed tomography) study is a hybridization of a standard medical maxillofacial CT scan and dental imaging. The CBCT delivers significantly less radiation than a conventional CT of the same anatomical area. With the newer CBCT units and low-dose protocols, this technology can deliver less radiation then routine full-mouth dental surveys. The focal point of the CBCT can be as small as .3 mm, which increases image clarity. It is recommended that these studies include a radiology report from a licensed radiologist. Whether the clinician is treating an airway problem or a jaw-function disorder, a CBCT study is indicated for optimal patient information.

Under all circumstances, whether treating airway or movement disorder problems involving the jaw, a CBCT study with radiology report is highly recommended.

General CBCT information:

- Degree of pharyngeal airway blockage and location of blockage
- Degree of nasal blockage
- Other pathology in the head, face, jaw, and neck area
- Degenerative joint disease (jaw joints and/or cervical spine)
- Posteriorly displaced mandibular condyles
- Abnormal joint anatomy
- Maxillomandibular orthognathic abnormalities
- Definitive evidence of dental and/or periodontal pathology

The literature provides guidelines for documenting the minimal cross-sectional area of the pharynx and risk factor for SDB/OSA. When the area is less than 52 mm^2, the risk for SDB/OSA is high; 52–110 mm^2, the risk is medium; and anything greater than 110 mm^2 has a mild risk for SDB/OSA.

Detailed CBCT information

1. Airway

   - Patency of airway
   - Location of narrowest aspect
   - Existence of growths, anatomical variations, or other pathology

2. Patient photographs

   - Symmetry
   - Anomalies

3. Jaw joints with lateral and frontal perspective (closed posture)

- Condyle location in fossa
- Condition of condyle and fossa

4. Lateral cephalometric (baseline anatomical comparison to norms)

   - Modified Sassouni analysis
   - Modified Steiner analysis
   - Hyoid positioning

5. Frontal cephalometric (baseline anatomical comparison to norms)

   - Grummons analysis

6. Sinuses

   - Patency
   - Existence of growths, anatomical variations, or other pathology

7. Nasal Airway

   - Condition of septum
   - Condition of internal soft tissue
   - Patency of airway
   - Existence of growths, anatomical variations, or other pathology

8. Dentition and alveolar support

   - Evidence of bone loss (periodontal disease)
   - Evidence of dental disease
   - Anomalies/pathology

9. Maxilla, mandible, and cervical spine

   - Anomalies/pathology

10. General

    - Anomalies/pathology

CHAPTER 7

Therapy for Sleep-Related Breathing and Movement Disorders

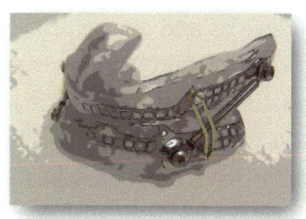

G enerally, therapy decisions for diagnosed sleep-related breathing disorders, specifically obstructive sleep apnea (OSA), are based upon their effectiveness in eliminating OSA events. Therapies for diagnosed movement disorders, specifically periodic limb movement disorder (PLMD), are based upon effectiveness in decreasing sleep-period muscle activity associated with arousals. The different forms of therapy include the following:

- Positive airway pressure (PAP)
- Mandibular repositioning device (MRD)
- Otolaryngological surgery
- Oral Maxillofacial surgery
- Medication

PAP devices provide a pneumatic splint to maintain an open airway. The PAP device creates pressurized airflow that is delivered through a facial mask or nasal cannula. There are five types of PAP devices:

1. Continuous positive airway pressure (CPAP)
2. Auto-adjusting positive airway pressure (AutoPAP)
3. Bilevel positive airway pressure (BiPAP)
4. Oral positive airway pressure (OPAP)
5. Oral device mounted nasal PAP

Positive Airway Pressure

CPAP maintains a constant air pressure flow set by the sleep physician or sleep technologist. AutoPAP utilizes an electronic sensor that adjusts the air pressure flow depending on degree of airway patency. BiPAP allows for higher inspiratory pressure and lower expiratory pressure. All PAP devices are equipped with electronics that monitor compliance and measured levels of AHI/RDI. Data memory cards can be downloaded onto provider computers. All mask interfaces must be properly fitted to maintain optimal facial and nasal seals. In most cases, an oral lip seal is important to apparatus effectiveness. Compliance is a recurrent problem with PAP, with patients noting claustrophobia, lack of facial or nasal seal, skin and eye irritation, and ingestion of air as causes of intolerance to the apparatus.

Mandibular Repositioning Device (MRD)

Mandibular repositioning devices (MRDs) are less effective in elimination of OSA events than PAP devices: however, compliance appears higher with oral devices and overall success of treatment may be relatively the same. Currently, research on compliance and efficacy monitoring for mandibular repositioning devices is underway. FDA-approved appliances—to maintain postural changes—come in a variety of designs using intraoral plastic, elastic arms, metal arms, metal screws, and hooks or bars. These devices achieve a more efficient airway by increasing tongue space, moving the tongue forward, artificially altering muscle tone, and altering tongue behavior. The major side effect of oral appliances is a long-term altered jaw posture, which can change the way the teeth meet. There is considerable crossover between the treatment of obstructive sleep apnea with mandibular repositioning devices and the treatment of temporomandibular disorders with orthotics and anterior repositioning appliances. Treatment strategies include the effective management of related OSA and TMD musculoskeletal issues. Follow-up sleep studies are necessary for comprehensive care.

Soft Tissue Surgery

Soft tissue and limited osseous surgery are generally provided by the otolaryngologist. These surgeries focus primarily on soft tissue reduction and removal. Surgeries include septoplasty, turbinate reduction, nasal polypectomy, tonsillectomy, uvulapalatopharyngoplasty, tongue base suspension and surgical reduction of the tongue. In selected cases, clinicians reposition the hyoid bone with hyoid suspension and reposition the tongue with genioglossus-advancement surgery. In severe, life-threatening cases, the entire airway can be bypassed and a tracheostomy performed. Surgical side effects are primarily the uncomfortable postsurgical experience, changes in oropharyngeal sensation, and food displacement into the nasopharynx. Surgery is considered less effective treatment, but is beneficial in selected cases. A follow-up sleep study is necessary for efficacy assessment.

Osseous Surgery

Hard tissue surgery is generally provided by the oral maxillofacial surgeon and specialized otolaryngologists. These procedures focus on maxillary and mandibular osteotomies, both of which require significant post-operative recovery periods. Side effects can include persistent pain and numbness. Positive outcomes have been reported with careful patient selection. Oral appliance pre-treatment may aid surgical planning.

Medication

Physician diagnosis may include periodic limb movement disorder (PLMD). This diagnosis suggests that sleep disruption and arousal with daytime somnolence are related to body movements observed during sleep studies. PLMD may occur alone or along with obstructive sleep disorders. Customary treatment involves either dopamine agonist, anti convulsant, sedative or opioid medication.

CHAPTER 8

Practice Management

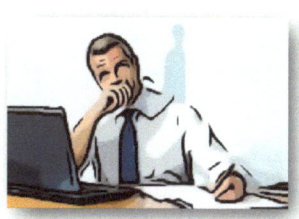

As dentists take on new responsibilities, their practices must adopt new models of management—a variety of which have been proposed in order to incorporate medical functions. Dentists who are exploring adding sleep medicine into their practices can be overwhelmed by the extensive, and often conflicting, information. Choosing the appropriate model that best fits the individual dental practice can be both time consuming and costly. Review of the literature, malpractice insurance, and state board guidelines is an important first step in the decision process.

In order to provide medical services within a dental practice, the dentist may provide educational pamphlets and simple screening devices to identify potential patients. If a patient is identified with symptoms consistent with sleep apnea, the dentist then refers the patient to the primary care physician (PCP) or sleep medicine specialist for diagnosis. The referral includes a face-to-face encounter with the physician along with a sleep study if the physician deems it appropriate. In some cases, the dentist may refer the patient directly for a sleep study. Oral-appliance titration versus CPAP titration during the sleep study can be requested. A board-certified sleep physician interprets the sleep study and may be involved in further workup of the patient.

Whether the patient is diagnosed with benign snoring or obstructive sleep apnea, the patient may be referred back to the dentist. If an oral appliance is considered as a potentially viable treatment, a prescription is written by the physician, requesting oral-appliance evaluation and care. Included with the referral and diagnosis are related medical records. The dentist should expect to receive clinical documentation of the diagnosis and a current copy of the sleep study.

The dentist who elects to treat snoring and obstructive sleep disorders is obligated to utilize current medical coding and billing practices. The *ICD-9/10* diagnosis protocol and *CPT/HCPCS* treatment codes are required.

Throughout the diagnostic and treatment process, Centers for Medicare and Medicaid Services (CMS) billing guidelines are generally followed.

Following recommended protocol requires an investment in the following:

- Medical billing system/module
- Medical records system/module
- Protocols for interfacing with physicians and medical offices
- The addition of staff (optional depending on office dynamics)

The immediate opportunity for dental providers to treat sleep-related breathing disorders exists within their own patient base. It is commonly expected that dentists screen their patient base while they begin marketing and developing patient awareness within the community.

Remuneration models for oral-appliance services vary in design:

- The dental provider may choose to assume economic risk and bill insurance directly, as an out-of-network provider.
- The dental provider may consider contracting directly with medical insurance carriers for payment on negotiated rates.
- The dental provider may contract with a third-party billing service for all related medical billing.
- The dental provider may adopt the fee-for-service model.
- The dental provider may adopt a hybrid model that combines aspects of the various options.

Regardless of the remuneration model, dental providers must adopt new levels of correspondence with medical insurance carriers, medical providers, and diagnostic laboratories.

Dental providers must also adopt current and consistent medical-patient records and documentation so that they can correspond and communicate meaningful clinical information to the following:

- Insurance carriers
- Physician groups
- Medical providers
- Diagnostic and appliance laboratories
- Dental colleagues

There are a variety of business philosophies, resources, and services that are available to dentists seeking expansion into the medical model of care. It is a matter of choosing the appropriate practice management model that meets the dentist's patient and practice needs.

CHAPTER 9

Sleep Medicine Terminology

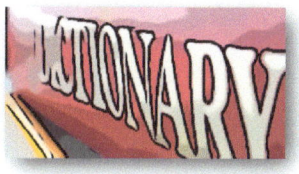

Advanced sleep phase syndrome: A change in sleep dynamics in which the sleep-wake cycle is advanced in a twenty-four-hour period.

Ambulatory sleep study or home sleep test (HST): Portable system used to record multiple physiological variables during sleep.

Anticonvulsants: Drugs that prevent or reduce the severity and frequency of seizures in various types of epilepsy

Apnea index (AI): A measure of the severity of sleep apnea by tracking the number of apnea events per hour.

Apnea-hypopnea index (AHI): The number of obstructive apnea and hypopnea events per hour of total sleep period.

Arousal: The abrupt change from sleep to wakefulness or from a deeper to lighter stage of sleep. These changes are recorded as an increase in EEG activity (arousal). An arousal may be accompanied by increase in muscle or heart activity. A documented arousal must have a duration of at least three seconds. Types of arousal are respiratory related, muscle activity or movement related, or spontaneous.

Arousal index: The number of arousals per hour of sleep period. Also called *sleep fragmentation*.

Arrhythmia: An irregular heartbeat resulting in tachycardia or bradycardia.

Atonia: A type of temporary muscle paralysis, as seen in REM sleep.

Attention deficit hyperactivity disorder (ADHD): Patients with ADHD have difficulty focusing on tasks and concentrating on one thing. Variants on this disorder include hyperactivity and hypoactivity.

Auto-adjusting positive airway pressure device (APAP): A type of PAP machine that monitors changes in breathing and adjusts automatically with variable pressure flow.

Benzodiazepines: A class of tranquilizing and sedating compounds used to enhance sleep and treat movement disorders.

Bi-level positive airway pressure device (BiPAP): A PAP device that is modified to provide a lower pressure for exhalation and a higher pressure for inhalation.

Body sleep posture: The four sleep positions: back (supine), left side, right side, or abdomen (prone). The time spent sleeping in each position and the number of respiratory events in a particular position is recorded.

Body mass index (BMI): A measurement of body fat based on height and weight that applies to both men and women. BMI can be used to determine whether patients are overweight, obese, underweight, or normal weight. A BMI score between twenty and twenty-five is considered normal; below twenty is considered underweight; and above twenty-five is considered overweight.

Bradycardia: A heart rhythm with a rate lower than sixty beats per minute.

Bruxism: The occurrence of abnormal muscle activity involving the jaw that may be static or involve muscle movement.

Cataplexy: A sudden, dramatic decrease in muscle control and loss of deep reflexes that follows a strong emotional or physical stimulus such as laughter, surprise, or sudden physical exercise, and is one of the tetrad of narcolepsy symptoms.

Central sleep apnea/hypopnea: Interruption of oral/nasal airflow not associated with respiratory effort or airway blockage; thought to be related to a temporary irregularity in the brain's control of breathing.

Cheyne–Stokes respiration (periodic breathing): An abnormal breathing pattern typified by crescendo-decrescendo or waxing and waning fluctuations in respiratory rate and tidal volume usually associated with congestive heart failure and neurological disease.

Circadian rhythm disorder: A change in the innate behavioral and physiological functions that affect sleeping and waking states within the normal twenty-four-hour cycle.

Cone-beam computed tomography (CBCT): The use of divergent, cone-shaped imaging of the head and neck that acquires volumetric data sets of nearly six hundred distinct images. The scanning software collects the data and reconstructs it, producing three-dimensional anatomical images that can be manipulated and viewed with specialized software.

Continuous positive airway pressure (CPAP): The device used to treat sleep apnea by creating continuous, positive airway pressure to maintain an open airway, enabling normal breathing through the patient's nose or mouth.

Craniomandibular cervical disorder (CMCD): A musculoskeletal imbalance that causes pain in the face, jaw, and neck. This condition may be associated with abnormal muscle activity and sleep disruption. Temporomandibular joint and upper-cervical degenerative changes have been observed.

Deep sleep: Stage 3 non-REM sleep associated with delta waves on electroencephalogram (EEG) recordings.

Delayed sleep phase: The sleep period is moved back in time within the customary sleep-wake cycle, resulting in a delayed occurrence of sleep within the twenty-four-hour period.

Delta sleep: The stage of sleep in which EEG delta waves are prevalent or predominant (non-REM-sleep stage 3).

Diagnostic sleep study: Used to monitor several physiological activities while the patient sleeps, it is commonly performed to determine the absence or presence of a specific sleep disorder. The sleep study may occur in a sleep-disorder center, or in a patient's home using portable recording equipment.

Diaphragm: The large, concave muscle attached to the rib cage at the bottom of the chest (top of the abdomen). Inhalation occurs when the diaphragm contracts and exhalation occurs when the diaphragm relaxes.

Diurnal: Indicates daytime activity versus nocturnal or nighttime activity.

Dopamine agonist: One of the main drugs indicated for treatment of Parkinson's like symptoms.

Durable medical equipment (DME): Prescribed healthcare equipment including positive airway pressure machines and mandibular repositioning devices.

Drowsiness: The patient has difficulty staying awake.

Electrocardiogram (EKG): A method of recording the heart's electrical activity that is used to document abnormal heart function including arrhythmia, tachycardia, and bradycardia.

Electroencephalogram (EEG): A method of recording the brain's electrical activity that is used to document sleep stages, arousals, and awakenings.

Electromyogram (EMG): A method of recording electrical activity from the muscular system that is used to document sleep stages, arousals, and awakenings. Surface electrodes are routinely placed on the submental jaw area. During REM sleep, the chin EMG is tonically inhibited. Electrodes may also be placed in the masseter and anterior temporalis muscle areas to record both jaw movement and muscle activity.

Electrooculogram (EOG): A recording of voltage changes resulting from shifts in position of the eyeball that is used to document sleep stages, arousals, and awakenings. Surface electrodes are placed near the eyes to record eyeball movement. Rapid eye movement characterizes the REM-sleep stage.

Epoch: A baseline thirty-second duration of a sleep recording.

Epworth Sleepiness Scale (ESS): Eight-question, self-reported survey of patient's propensity to fall asleep during the day. A score of seven or above is considered elevated.

Excessive daytime sleepiness or somnolence (EDS): A subjective patient's report documenting their difficulty in staying awake during the day.

Fatigue: A feeling of tiredness or weariness during waking hours.

Fiber-optic nasopharyngoscope: A flexible fiber-optic scope used to examine nasal passages, nasopharynx, oropharynx, and laryngopharynx.

Fibromyalgia: An idiopathic syndrome characterized by primary symptoms of multiple areas of muscle pain and feelings of fatigue.

Gastroesophageal reflux disease (GERD): An abnormal flow of stomach acid upward into the esophagus associated with noxious taste, arousals, and disrupted sleep.

Genioglossus advancement: A surgical procedure used for sleep apnea or snoring. A segment of mandibular symphysis containing the anterior attachment of the genioglossus muscle is pulled forward and stabilized, posturing the tongue more forward and preventing it from blocking the airway.

Heart rate (beats per minute): The pace or speed of the heart measured in beats per minute. Sixty to eighty beats per minute is considered a normal heart rate in adults.

Hertz (Hz): A measure of sound frequency in cycles per second (cps).

Hyoid suspension: A surgical procedure used in the treatment of sleep apnea or snoring. The hyoid bone is located in the neck, anterior to the airway, with multiple muscle attachments. The hyoid bone is pulled forward and downward and is attached to the superior aspect of the thyroid cartilage, opening the airway.

Hypercapnia: An elevated level of carbon dioxide in the blood.

Hypersomnia: An excessive, prolonged duration of sleep.

Hypertension: Abnormally high blood pressure.

Hypnotics: Psychoactive drugs with a primary function of inducing sleep, used as a treatment for insomnia.

Hypoventilation: A reduced rate and depth of breathing.

Hypoxemia: A reduced level of oxygen in the blood.

Hypoxia: Occurs when insufficient oxygen reaches the tissues of the body.

Imidazopyridines: A class of compounds used to induce sleepiness such as Zolpidem, which goes by the trade name Ambien.

Insomnia: Difficulty falling asleep (initiation insomnia), or difficulty maintaining the sleep state (maintenance insomnia), associated with sleep loss.

Laryngopharynx: The lower portion of the pharynx extending from the tip of the epiglottis to the larynx.

Laser assisted uvulopalatoplasty (LAUP): The laser ablation of excessive palatal soft tissue used to reduce snoring and sleep apnea.

Light sleep: A term used to describe non-REM-sleep stages 1 and 2.

Light therapy: A modality used in the treatment of seasonal affective disorder (SAD). This therapy exposes the eyes to light of appropriate intensity and duration and at the appropriate time of day to affect the timing, duration, and quality of sleep.

Macroglossia: An overly large tongue.

Maintenance of wakefulness test (MWT): A measure of an individual's degree of alertness during waking hours. Maintenance of wakefulness testing is indicated when the individual's ability to remain awake becomes a personal or professional safety issue. Mean sleep latencies that are less than eight minutes are considered abnormal.

Mandibular repositioning device (MRD): An intraoral device used to treat obstructive sleep disorders and snoring. The device is normally secured by the dentition, and is designed to reposition the mandible anteriorly and vertically, bringing the tongue forward, maintaining an open airway.

Maxillomandibular orthotic (MMO): An intraoral device used to treat temporomandibular disorders. This therapy is focused on altering neuromuscular patterns and improving jaw area muscle and joint function. The device is designed to reposition the mandible anteriorly, laterally, vertically and in some cases, allowing rotational changes. Also called a mandibular anterior repositioning appliance (MARA) or anterior repositioning appliance (ARA).

Maxillofacial: A term that refers to the anatomical area of the middle and lower face and the jaws.

Maxillomandibular osteotomy and advancement (MMOA): A surgical procedure developed for patients with retro-lingual airway obstruction. The procedure involves the surgical fracturing and postural advancement of the maxilla and mandible or is limited to advancement of the mandible only.

Mixed sleep apnea: A complete absence of airflow for more than ten seconds accompanied by a complete absence of respiratory effort (central apnea) at the beginning of the event followed by a gradual increase in effort (obstructive apnea) over time.

Movement arousal: Body movement associated with arousal or awakening.

Multiple sleep latency test (MSLT): A series of nap tests utilized to assess excessive daytime sleepiness (narcolepsy).

Muscle tone: The amount of tension and contraction in a muscle.

Myoclonus: Muscle contractions in the form of jerks or twitches.

Narcolepsy: A sleep disorder characterized by excessive sleepiness, cataplexy, sleep paralysis, hallucinations, and a tendency to pass directly from wakefulness into REM sleep.

Nasal airflow/nasal ventilation: A pressure recording (thermistor) of the complete respiratory cycle by measuring inspiratory and expiratory airflow.

Nasal speculum: A medical tool for investigating patency of the nasal airway.

Neurotransmitters: The endogenous biochemicals that are released from axon terminals of one neuron and transmit the signal to the next neuron by combining with its receptor molecules. Neurotransmitters important in the control of sleep and wakefulness include: norepinephrine, serotonin, acetylcholine, dopamine, adrenaline, and histamine.

Nocturia: Excessive, often frequent, urination during the night.

Nocturnal: The patient demonstrates high levels of activity during the dark, customary sleep period. See also *diurnal*.

Nocturnal confusion: Episodes of delirium or disorientation near or during nighttime sleep; often seen in the elderly, and patients suffering from Alzheimer's disease.

Nocturnal penile tumescence (NPT): The hardening and expansion of the penis during sleep (penile erection) associated with nocturnal arousal.

Non-REM sleep (NREM): The three stages of sleep not characterized by rapid eye movement. These stages progress from lighter to deeper sleep (stages 1 through 3).

Obstructive sleep apnea/hypopnea: Airway blockage resulting in interruption in oral/nasal airflow for 10 seconds or more, ranging from partial to full cessation of breathing accompanied by respiratory effort, arousal from sleep level, decrease in blood oxygen.

Opioids: Primary use of this category of drug is to obtund pain with side effect of sedation.

Oral appliance therapy (OAT): Non-specific term for treatment of multiple jaw related disorders with an oral appliance.

Oxygen desaturation: A condition that reflects a decrease in the amount of oxygen carried by hemoglobin in the blood; values below 90 percent are considered abnormal.

Oxygen saturation: A measure of the oxygen carried by hemoglobin in the blood; normal values are 90 to 100 percent.

Oximeter (pulse): An instrument that provides estimates of arterial oxyhemoglobin saturation (SaO2) by utilizing selected wavelengths of light to determine the saturation of oxyhemoglobin (SpO2). The sensor is usually attached to the finger.

Parasomnia: A number of abnormal conditions that occur during sleep such as sleep- walking, sleep-talking, bruxing, and clenching.

Paroxysmal nocturnal dyspnea (PND): Respiratory distress and shortness of breath due to pulmonary edema that often awakens the sleeping individual.

Periodic limb movement disorder (PLMD): A condition characterized by periodic episodes of repetitive limb movements occurring during sleep. The muscle activity and movements are associated with arousals and awakenings.

PLMD index: The number of sleep-related limb movements per hour of sleep.

PLMD arousal index: The number of sleep-related limb movements per hour of sleep that are associated with an arousal (more than fifteen per hour is considered significant).

Pharynx: The area posterior to the nose and the oral cavity extending from the base of the skull to the larynx that functions as the passageway for air. Also, partially used for food and liquid ingestion from the mouth to the esophagus.

Physical medicine: The branch of medicine that focuses on enhancing and restoring physical capabilities to those with physical impairments or disabilities.

Pineal gland: The gland in the brain that secretes the hormone melatonin.

Polysomnogram (PSG): The continuous and simultaneous recording of physiological variables during sleep. Basic physiologic measures include EEG, EOG, EMG, EKG, respiratory air flow, and limb and jaw movement. Used primarily for the diagnosis of sleep-related breathing and movement disorders.

Positive airway pressure (PAP): A mode of respiratory ventilation used primarily in the treatment of sleep apnea. The pressure needed to maintain an open airway in a sleep apnea patient expressed in centimeters of water displacement (cm H2O). The positive pressure can range from five to twenty centimeters H2O according to patient requirements as determined by a CPAP titration study.

Radio frequency ablation (RF): A surgical procedure also known as *somnoplasty* for reducing nasal and oropharyngeal soft tissue thought to be involved in airway obstruction.

REM sleep: A sleep stage characterized by rapid eye movement, increased brain activity, and muscle atonia; most dreaming occurs in this stage, which accounts for approximately 20 percent of sleep in adults.

REM motor atonia: The suppression of voluntary muscle activity during REM sleep.

Respiratory disturbance index (RDI): The total of obstructive apneas, hypopneas, and respiratory effort-related arousals divided by total hours of sleep time.

Respiratory events: The total number of obstructive, mixed, and central apneas and hypopneas, plus respiratory effort-related arousals.

Respiratory effort-related arousal (RERA): Breathing disorder characterized by obstructed upper airway with airflow reduction which does not meet the criteria of apnea or hypopnea, associated with increase in respiratory effort accompanied by arousal from sleep level.

Restless leg or limb syndrome (RLS): A sleep disorder characterized by a deep creeping or crawling sensation in the legs that occurs when an individual is awake and sedentary. The sensations are often relieved by movement.

Sagittal: The side view of the face (lateral perspective). Similar terminology for other axes of the human body would include axial for the vertical perspective and coronal for the anterior/posterior perspective. Synonyms for sagittal/axial/coronal are lateral/frontal/superior-inferior.

Septoplasty: A surgery on the nasal septum to enhance airflow.

Sleep: A state marked by lessened consciousness, lessened movement of the skeletal muscles, and slowed-down metabolism.

Sleep apnea event: A near to complete cessation of oral/nasal airflow for 10 seconds or more with an accompanying decrease in blood oxygen and arousal from sleep level.

Sleep architecture: Non-REM-sleep stages 1–3 and REM-sleep stage. These stages cycle four to six times throughout the sleep period. Of the total sleep time, 75–80 percent is typically NREM, and 20–25 percent is REM stage sleep (NREM stage 1: 10 percent; stage 2: 50 percent; stage 3: 20 percent; and REM: 20 percent total sleep time/TST).

Sleep cycle: A progression of sleep states from lighter (stages 1 and 2) to deeper sleep (stage 3) levels. Stages 1–3 are considered non-REM sleep, and there is only one stage of REM sleep. The sleep states continue to alternate throughout the night with an average period of about approximately 90 ninety minutes. A night of normal sleep typically consists of four to six cycles.

Sleep debt: The result of recurrent sleep deprivation that occurs over time when an individual has an insufficient amount of the restorative daily sleep that is required to feel rested and refreshed.

Sleep deprivation: An acute or chronic lack of sufficient sleep.

Sleep disorders: A broad range of possible health problems arising from numerous causes including dysfunctional sleep mechanisms, abnormalities in physiological functions during sleep, abnormalities of the biological clock, and sleep disturbances that are induced by factors extrinsic to the sleep process.

Sleep efficiency (SE): The proportion of sleep during the designated sleep period; the ratio of total sleep time to total time spent in bed.

Sleep fragmentation: Clinical evidence of sleep disruption with arousals occurring throughout the night, reducing the total amount of time spent in the deeper levels of sleep.

Sleep hygiene: Those conditions and practices that promote continuous and effective sleep including: regulating bedtime and waking times; adjusting time spent in bed to the time necessary for sustained and adequate sleep (i.e., the total sleep time sufficient to avoid sleepiness when awake); restricting alcohol and caffeine intake in the period prior to bedtime; and adjusting exercise, nutritional, and environmental factors so that they enhance, rather than disturb, restful sleep.

Sleep hyperhidrosis: Excessive sweating during sleep associated with hormonal changes; the condition may be responsible for arousals.

Sleep hypopnea event: A partial interruption in oral/nasal airflow for ten seconds or more with an accompanying decrease in blood oxygen and arousal from sleep level.

Sleep latency: The time period measured from actual bedtime to the beginning of the sleep state. Used to support diagnoses of narcolepsy (excessive daytime sleepiness), EDS, cataplexy, hypnagogic hallucinations, and sleep paralysis.

Sleep mentations: The thoughts, feelings, images, perceptions, hallucinations, and active dreams occurring during sleep that may diminish the quality of sleep.

Sleep-related breathing disorder (SRBD): The term refers to the spectrum of breathing anomalies ranging from chronic or habitual snoring to upper airway resistance syndrome to central and obstructive sleep apnea.

Sleep stages: Sleep stages are cyclical rather than linear. Sleep begins in stage 1 and progresses into stages 2 and 3. After stage 3 sleep, stage 2 sleep may be repeated before entering REM sleep. Once REM sleep is over, the body usually returns to stage 2 sleep. Sleep cycles through these stages approximately four or five times throughout the night. On average, we enter the REM stage approximately ninety minutes after falling asleep. The first cycle of REM sleep might last only a short amount of time, but each cycle becomes longer. REM sleep can last up to an hour as sleep progresses.

Sleep stage 1: The beginning of the sleep cycle; a relatively light stage of sleep. Stage 1 can be considered a transition period between wakefulness and sleep. In stage 1, the brain produces high-amplitude theta waves, which are very slow brain waves. This period of sleep lasts approximately 5 percent of total sleep time.

Sleep stage 2: The second stage of sleep lasts for approximately twenty minutes. The brain begins to produce bursts of rapid, rhythmic brain wave activity known as sleep spindles. Body temperature decreases and heart rate slows. This period of sleep lasts approximately 50 percent of total sleep time.

Sleep stage 3: This stage was previously divided into stages 3 and 4. Deep, slow brain waves known as delta waves emerge during stage 3 sleep; this stage is sometimes referred to as delta, or slow-wave, sleep. During this stage, people become less responsive and noises and activity in the environment may fail to generate a response. It also acts as a transitional period between light sleep and very deep sleep. Bed-wetting and sleepwalking are most likely to occur at the end of this stage of sleep. This sleep period comprises approximately 25 percent of total sleep time.

Sleep stage REM: Most dreaming occurs during the fourth stage of sleep, known as rapid eye movement (REM) sleep. REM sleep is characterized by eye movement, increased respiration rate, and increased brain activity. REM sleep is also referred to as paradoxical sleep because while activity in the brain and other body systems increases, the muscles become more relaxed. Dreaming occurs, along with increased brain activity and paralysis of voluntary musculature. Stage REM is approximately 20 percent of total sleep time.

Snoring: The sound produced by the vibration of respiratory structures as a result of obstructed air movement during the sleep period.

Stanford Sleepiness Scale (SSS): Rating scale consisting of seven numbered statements describing subjective levels of sleepiness and alertness.

Temporomandibular disorder (TMD): A musculoskeletal imbalance involving the jaw joints and surrounding musculature. Symptoms vary from jaw-area discomfort to jaw-joint noises and restricted muscle activity. TMD is often found as a comorbidity in obstructive sleep apnea patients. Abnormal muscle activity with clenching, excessive jaw movement, and sleep disruption has been observed.

Temporomandibular joint (TMJ): The bilateral articulation between the base of the skull and the mandible. A diarthrodial joint that allows both rotational and translational function.

Tachycardia: A condition of rapid heart rate, usually defined by a pulse rate of over one hundred beats per minute.

Tongue-retaining device (TRD): A pliable intraoral device that holds the tongue forward using a tongue compartment and suction. The device has been used on patients who are edentulous, and who have a limited range of motion. This appliance is not appropriate for mouth breathers.

Total sleep time (TST): The amount of actual sleep time within a sleep period, calculated by total sleep period less arousal and waking time.

Tracheotomy: A surgical procedure that creates an opening in the trachea so that the patient can breathe.

Tracheostomy: The actual opening in the trachea that is created by surgery. This opening is normally enhanced with plastic tubing.

Tricyclic antidepressants: A medication for the treatment of depression and to control cataplectic attacks, hypnogogic hallucinations, and sleep paralysis. Most tricyclic antidepressants also reduce REM sleep.

Turbinates: The small, shelf-like cartilaginous structures covered by mucous membranes that protrude into the nasal airway to help warm, humidify, and cleanse inhaled air on its way to the lungs.

Upper airway resistance syndrome (UARS): A part of the spectrum of obstructive sleep-related breathing disorders in which repetitive increases in resistance to airflow in the upper airway lead to arousals and daytime fatigue. Apneas and hypopneas may be totally absent. Blood-oxygen levels can be in the normal range.

Uvula: The small, soft structure hanging from the bottom of the soft palate in the midline above the back of the tongue.

Uvulopalatopharyngoplasty (UPPP): Surgery to reduce the tissue of the soft palate, uvula, and pharyngeal tonsil area.

CHAPTER 10

Recommended Reading and Oral Appliance Research

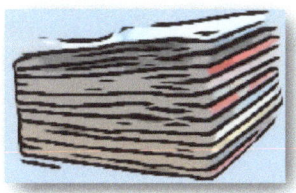

Recommended Reading

Bruxism: Theory and Practice (Paesani)

Dental Management of Sleep Disorders (Attanasio and Bailey)

Principles and Practice of Sleep Medicine (Kryger, Roth, and Dement)

Sleep Medicine and Dentistry (Attanasio and Bailey, ed. *Dental Clinics of North America* Vol. 56, No. 2, 2012.)

Sleep Medicine for Dentists: A Practical Overview (Lavigne, Cistulli, and Smith)

Snoring and Obstructive Sleep Apnea (Fairbanks and Woodson)

Somnology (T. Lee-Chiong)

The Integrated Dental Medical System (Chase)

Oral Appliance Research

- Ferguson, K. A., et al., Oral Appliances for Snoring and Obstructive Sleep Apnea: a Review. Sleep, 2006. 29(2): p. 244–62.
- Scherr S. C, D. L., Almeida F. R, Bennett K. M, Blumenstock N. T, Demko B. G, Essick G. K, Katz S. G, McLornan P. M, Phillips and P. R. K. S, Rogers R. R, Schell T. G, Sheats R. D, Sreshta F. P., Definition of an Effective Oral Appliance for the Treatment of Obstructive Sleep Apnea and Snoring: a Report of the American Academy of Dental Sleep Medicine. Journal of Dental Sleep Medicine, 2014. 1(1): p. 39–50.
- Gauthier, L., et al., Efficacy of Two Mandibular Advancement Appliances in the Management of Snoring and Mild-Moderate Sleep Apnea: a Cross-over Randomized Study. Sleep Med, 2009. 10(3): p. 329–36.
- Gauthier, L., et al., Mandibular Advancement Appliances Remain Effective in Lowering Respiratory Disturbance Index for 2.5–4.5 years. Sleep Med, 2011. 12(9): p. 844–9.
- Gotsopoulos, H., et al., Oral Appliance Therapy Improves Symptoms in Obstructive Sleep Apnea: a Randomized, Controlled Trial. Am J Respir Crit Care Med, 2002. 166(5): p. 743–8.
- Holley, A. B., C. J. Lettieri, and A. A. Shah, Efficacy of an Adjustable Oral Appliance and Comparison with Continuous Positive Airway Pressure for the Treatment of Obstructive Sleep Apnea Syndrome. Chest, 2011. 140(6): p. 1511–6
- Randerath, W. J., et al., An Individually Adjustable Oral Appliance vs Continuous Positive Airway Pressure in Mild-to-Moderate Obstructive Sleep Apnea Syndrome. Chest, 2002. 122(2): p. 569–75.
- Qaseem, A., et al., Management of Obstructive Sleep Apnea in Adults: A Clinical Practice Guideline From the American College of Physicians. Ann Intern Med, 2013.
- Epstein, L. J., et al., Clinical Guideline for the Evaluation, Management and Long-Term Care of Obstructive Sleep Apnea in Adults. J Clin Sleep Med, 2009. 5(3): p. 263–76.
- Johnston, C. D., et al., Mandibular Advancement Appliances and Obstructive Sleep Apnoea: a Randomized Clinical Trial. Eur J Orthod, 2002. 24(3): p. 251–62.
- Cooke, M. E. and J. M. Battagel, A Thermoplastic Mandibular Advancement Device for the Management of Non-Apnoeic Snoring: a Randomized Controlled Trial. Eur J Orthod, 2006. 28(4): p. 32–38.
- Robertson, S., et al., A Randomized Crossover Trial of Conservative Snoring Treatments: Mandibular Repositioning Splint and Nasal CPAP. Otolaryngol Head Neck Surg, 2008. 138(3): p. 283–288.
- Aarab, G., et al., Oral Appliance Therapy Versus Nasal Continuous Positive Airway Pressure in Obstructive Sleep Apnea: a Randomized, Placebo-Controlled Trial. Respiration, 2011. 81(5): p. 411–9.
- Aarab, G., et al., Long-Term Follow-Up of a Randomized Controlled Trial of Oral Appliance Therapy in Obstructive Sleep Apnea. Respiration, 2011. 82(2): p. 162–8.
- Barnes, M., et al., Efficacy of Positive Airway Pressure and Oral Appliance in Mild to Moderate Obstructive Sleep Apnea. Am J Respir Crit Care Med, 2004. 170(6): p. 656–64.
- Blanco, J., et al., Prospective Evaluation of an Oral Appliance in the Treatment of Obstructive Sleep Apnea Syndrome. Sleep Breath, 2005. 9(1): p. 20–5.
- Campbell, A. J., et al., Mandibular Advancement Splint Titration in Obstructive Sleep Apnoea. Sleep Breath, 2009. 13(2): p. 157–62.

- Cunali, P. A., et al., Mandibular Exercises Improve Mandibular Advancement Device Therapy for Obstructive Sleep Apnea. Sleep Breath, 2011. 15(4): p. 717–27.
- Deane, S. A., et al., Comparison of Mandibular Advancement Splint and Tongue Stabilizing Device in Obstructive Sleep Apnea: a Randomized Controlled Trial. Sleep, 2009. 32(5): p. 648–53.
- Ferguson, K. A., et al., A Randomized Crossover Study of an Oral Appliance vs Nasal-Continuous Positive Airway Pressure in the Treatment of Mild-Moderate Obstructive Sleep Apnea. Chest, 1996. 109(5): p. 1269–75.
- Gagnadoux, F., et al., Titrated Mandibular Advancement Versus Positive Airway Pressure for Sleep Apnoea. Eur Respir J, 2009. 34(4): p. 914–20.
- Ghazal, A., et al., A Randomized Prospective Long-Term Study of Two Oral Appliances for Sleep Apnoea Treatment. J Sleep Res, 2009. 18(3): p. 321–8.
- Gotsopoulos, H., J. J. Kelly, and P. A. Cistulli, Oral Appliance Therapy Reduces Blood Pressure in Obstructive Sleep Apnea: a Randomized, Controlled Trial. Sleep, 2004. 27(5): p. 934–41.
- Hoekema, A., et al., Simulated Driving in Obstructive Sleep Apnoea-Hypopnoea; Effects of Oral Appliances and Continuous Positive Airway Pressure. Sleep Breath, 2007. 11(3): p. 129–38.
- Hoekema, A., et al., Sexual Function and Obstructive Sleep Apnea-Hypopnea: a Randomized Clinical Trial Evaluating the Effects of Oral-Appliance and Continuous Positive Airway Pressure therapy. J Sex Med, 2007. 4(4 Pt 2): p. 1153–62.
- Hoekema, A., et al., Obstructive Sleep Apnea Therapy. J Dent Res, 2008. 87(9): p. 882–7.
- Hoekema, A., et al., Effects of Oral Appliances and CPAP on the Left Ventricle and Natriuretic Peptides. Int J Cardiol, 2008. 128(2): p. 232–9.
- Lawton, H. M., J. M. Battagel, and B. Kotecha, A Comparison of the Twin Block and Herbst Mandibular Advancement Splints in the Treatment of Patients with Obstructive Sleep Apnoea: a Prospective Study. Eur J Orthod, 2005. 27(1): p. 82–90.
- Mehta, A., et al., A Randomized, Controlled Study of a Mandibular Advancement Splint for Obstructive Sleep Apnea. Am J Respir Crit Care Med, 2001. 163(6): p. 1457–61.
- Naismith, S. L., et al., Effect of Oral Appliance Therapy on Neurobehavioral Functioning in Obstructive Sleep Apnea: a Randomized Controlled Trial. J Clin Sleep Med, 2005. 1(4): p. 374–80.
- Phillips, C. L., et al., Health Outcomes of Continuous Positive Airway Pressure Versus Oral Appliance Treatment for Obstructive Sleep Apnea: a Randomized Controlled Trial. Am J Respir Crit Care Med, 2013. 187(8): p. 879–87.
- Rose, E., et al., A Comparative Study of Two Mandibular Advancement Appliances for the Treatment of Obstructive Sleep Apnoea. Eur J Orthod, 2002. 24(2): p. 191–8.
- Sutherland, K., et al., Comparative Effects of Two Oral Appliances on Upper Airway Structure in Obstructive Sleep Apnea. Sleep, 2011. 34(4): p. 469–77.
- Tan, Y. K., et al., Mandibular Advancement Splints and Continuous Positive Airway Pressure in Patients with Obstructive Sleep Apnoea: a Randomized Cross-Over Trial. Eur J Orthod, 2002. 24(3): p. 239–49.
- Trzepizur, W., et al., Microvascular Endothelial Function in Obstructive Sleep Apnea: Impact of Continuous Positive Airway Pressure and Mandibular Advancement. Sleep Med, 2009. 10(7): p. 746–52.

- Vanderveken, O. M., et al., Comparison of a Custom-Made and a Thermoplastic Oral Appliance for the Treatment of Mild Sleep Apnea. Am J Respir Crit Care Med, 2008. 178(2): p. 197–202.
- Wilhelmsson, B., et al., A Prospective Randomized Study of a Dental Appliance Compared with Uvulopalatopharyngoplasty in the Treatment of Obstructive Sleep Apnoea. Acta Otolaryngol, 1999. 119(4): p. 503–9.
- Zhou, J. and Y. H. Liu, A Randomised Titrated Crossover Study Comparing Two Oral Appliances in the Treatment for Mild to Moderate Obstructive Sleep Apnoea/Hypopnoea Syndrome. J Oral Rehabil, 2012. 39(12): p. 914–22.
- Andren, A., et al., Effects of Treatment with Oral Appliance on 24-h Blood Pressure in Patients with Obstructive Sleep Apnea and Hypertension: a Randomized Clinical Trial. Sleep Breath, 2013. 17(2): p. 705–12.
- Doff, M. H., et al., Long-Term Oral Appliance Therapy in Obstructive Sleep Apnea Syndrome: a Controlled Study on Temporomandibular Side Effects. Clin Oral Investig, 2012. 16(3): p. 689–97.
- Doff, M. H., et al., Long-Term Oral Appliance Therapy in Obstructive Sleep Apnea Syndrome: a Controlled Study on Dental Side Effects. Clin Oral Investig, 2013. 17(2): p. 475–82.
- Lam, B., et al., Randomised Study of Three Non-Surgical Treatments in Mild to Moderate Obstructive Sleep Apnoea. Thorax, 2007. 62(4): p. 354–9.
- Doff, M. H., et al., Long-Term Oral-Appliance Therapy in Obstructive Sleep Apnea: a Cephalometric Study of Craniofacial Changes. J Dent, 2010. 38(12): p. 1010–8.
- Tsuda, H., et al., Craniofacial Changes After 2 Years of Nasal Continuous Positive Airway Pressure Use in Patients with Obstructive Sleep Apnea. Chest, 2010. 138(4): p. 870–4.
- Nieto, F. J., et al., Association of Sleep-Disordered Breathing, Sleep Apnea, and Hypertension in a Large Community-Based Study. Sleep Heart Health Study. JAMA, 2000. 283(14): p. 1829–36
- Silverberg, D. S., A. Oksenberg, and A. Iaina, Sleep-Related Breathing Disorders as a Major Cause of Essential Hypertension: Fact or Fiction? Curr Opin Nephrol Hypertens, 1998. 7(4): p. 353–7.
- Ferguson, K. A., et al., A Short-Term Controlled Trial of an Adjustable Oral Appliance for the Treatment of Mild to Moderate Obstructive Sleep Apnoea. Thorax, 1997. 52(4): p. 362–8.
- Engleman, H. M., et al., Randomized Crossover Trial of Two Treatments for Sleep Apnea/Hypopnea Syndrome: Continuous Positive Airway Pressure and Mandibular Repositioning Splint. Am J Respir Crit Care Med, 2002. 166(6): p. 855–9.
- Bloch, K. E., et al., A Randomized, Controlled Crossover Trial of Two Oral Appliances for Sleep Apnea Treatment. Am J Respir Crit Care Med, 2000. 162(1): p. 246–51.
- Clark, G. T., et al., A Crossover Study Comparing the Efficacy of Continuous Positive Airway Pressure with Anterior Mandibular Positioning Devices on Patients with Obstructive Sleep Apnea. Chest, 1996. 109(6): p. 1477–83.
- Kushida, C. A., et al., Practice Parameters for the Treatment of Snoring and Obstructive Sleep Apnea with Oral Appliances: an Update for 2005. Sleep, 2006. 29(2): p. 240–3.

About the Author

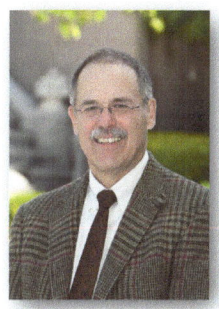

The Medical Dental Guild presents *Sleep Medicine and Oral Appliance Therapy*, a manual designed to assist both physicians and dentists as they consider active roles in the field of Sleep Medicine. Lead author, Dr. Peter Chase, DDS, MA is a past director of the Orofacial Disorders Center and professor at the University of the Pacific. He has a master's degree in education and extensive experience in multidisciplinary care for obstructive sleep apnea (OSA) and temporomandibular disorders (TMD). He has lectured widely, authored numerous articles, contributed to textbooks, published *The Integrated Medical Dental System (IDMS)*, and has proposed major changes to dental school curricula. He is currently in a private practice limited to OSA and TMD care. He maintains affiliations with multiple hospitals, medical groups, and sleep centers. Dr. Chase has served as a consultant to business, insurance, legal and professional organizations.